STUDYING
MIND-BODY HEALTH
AT COMMUNITY COLLEGES

TOWARD A COMPREHENSIVE
UNDERSTANDING OF HEALTH

EDITED BY
BARRY S. EISENBERG

This AACC publication was prepared
with funding from the Fetzer Institute.

American Association of Community Colleges
National Center for Higher Education
One Dupont Circle, NW, Suite 410
Washington, DC 20036
202/728-0200

© Copyrighted 1995
Printed in the United States
ISBN 0-87117-291-7

This publication was desktop published by Nadya Labib, Humanities
Program Associate, American Association of Community Colleges

TABLE OF CONTENTS

Part I

FOREWORD

DAVID R. PIERCE

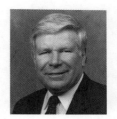

O n March 14-15, 1995, the American Association of Community Colleges and the Fetzer Institute, an education and research foundation based in Kalamazoo, Michigan, cosponsored a two-day roundtable of community college leaders with experience in the emerging field of mind-body health, and other experts working in this area. The roundtable participants met to examine ways in which the study of connections between our minds and bodies might be integrated into the community college curriculum. Their deliberations were guided by the results of a nationwide survey conducted by Katherine Bracey Lorenzo, Ph.D., to determine both the current status of mind-body studies on community college campuses and the degree of community college interest in this field for the future.

This publication is the result of their efforts. It is intended as an informational document for community colleges as they consider ways in which to respond to increased public interest in various forms of well-being. Included are suggestions offered to community colleges by the roundtable participants, a set of papers that introduce and elaborate on the meaning of mind-body health, results of the Lorenzo survey and a listing of mind-body health resources. It is, in effect, yet another "building community" resource. By expanding the spectrum of college offerings in the field of mind-body health, we are providing the communities we serve with an enhanced, more comprehensive understanding of health options.

The American Association of Community Colleges appreciates the support of the Fetzer Institute for this publication. It allows AACC to fulfill its traditional role of providing the nation's community colleges with awareness of new and cutting-

David R. Pierce is President and Chief Executive Officer of the American Association of Community Colleges.

edge areas of study. We are particularly indebted to the Fetzer Institute's David Sluyter for initiating this effort, to Diane U. Eisenberg for its execution and to Barry S. Eisenberg for producing this publication.

Part II

PREFACE

DAVID SLUYTER

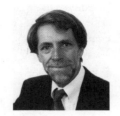

I n February of 1993, PBS aired a five-part series entitled *Healing and the Mind With Bill Moyers.* This series resulted in nearly unparalleled viewership for PBS and was influential in bringing the concepts of mind-body health to scientists, government officials, policy makers, and health professionals. In addition, it sparked the interest of thousands of people in communities all over the country. To meet this continuing interest, the Fetzer Institute felt that there was a need for accurate and easily available information and education in this area which has frequently been plagued by misinformation and exaggerated claims. It seemed like a natural need for community colleges to fill, given their interest in and outreach to the communities they serve and given their diverse student populations. Therefore, in March 1995, the Fetzer Institute and the American Association of Community Colleges (AACC) co-sponsored a roundtable to explore avenues for integrating mind-body health into the community college curriculum.

The roundtable was held at Seasons: A Center for Renewal, a retreat center at the Fetzer Institute which was built to bring people together in community and in dialogue. In this setting, twelve community college leaders, along with experts from the field of mind-body health, met to discuss the promise and potential of studies in mind-body health for community colleges, and also the potential barriers that may be encountered. The meeting began with presentations by James S. Gordon, M.D., a nationally acclaimed expert in the field of mind-body health, Molly Vass, Ed.D., Director of the Holistic Healthcare Program at Western Michigan University, and Katherine Bracey Lorenzo, Ph.D., who has been organizing mind-body health studies at Macomb Community College and had conducted

David Sluyter, Ed.D., is Program Director for Education at the Fetzer Institute.

a state-of-the-art survey of mind-body health programming at community colleges as part of this Fetzer Institute/AACC initiative. These presentations were followed by a day of dialogue and ended with the development of suggestions for community colleges, and the national organizations and foundations that share their educational concerns.

What follows are the results of this dialogue — a dialogue that will continue and expand in the months to follow. This publication can mark the beginning of a new way of thinking about health and wellness — about how people can use their minds to affect their bodies and begin to take control over and assume responsibility for their health. And it can help equip community colleges to begin to assume leadership roles in responding to the growing need on the part of the public for educational programs and courses in this emerging field. With this publication, we invite you to take part in this continuing discussion.

Part III

STUDYING MIND-BODY HEALTH AT COMMUNITY COLLEGES ...
TOWARD A COMPREHENSIVE UNDERSTANDING OF HEALTH

AACC/FETZER INSTITUTE ROUNDTABLE REPORT

"Health depends on a state of equilibrium among the various factors that govern the operation of the body and the mind; equilibrium, in turn, is reached only when man lives in harmony with his external environment."
Hippocrates, 460? - 377? B.C.

"Those [of us] who advocate educating the total personality point out that man's behavior is determined only in part by intellectual processes and decisions. Equally, if not more important are the emotions [and their connection to] physical and mental health."
B. Lamar Johnson, General Education in America, 1952

"Exploration is the key ... The journey [to understand the mind-body connection] is worth making for what each of us might learn about this remarkable union of mind, body and spirit that is the human being."
Bill Moyers, Healing and the Mind, 1993

WHAT IS MIND-BODY HEALTH?

For hundreds of years, Western philosophers and scientists have assumed that the mind and body are completely separate entities. Today this fundamental assumption is being challenged. The connections between mind and body are being studied in a broad range of research arenas. The relationship between these two spheres is being redefined, and a new basis for expanding the frontier of healing is being established.

Evidence is mounting that increased understanding of the mind-body connection may not only improve the quality of life, but actually affect the course of disease itself. A large number of new clinical studies are underway at leading U.S. medical institutions to measure the effects of mind-body techniques and to explore the physiological basis for these effects — studies to probe such questions as: "How do thoughts and feelings influence health?," "How is healing related to the mind?," and "What is health?" Examples of such studies include:

- University of Massachusetts Medical Center, where Jon Kabat-Zinn, Ph.D., associate professor of medicine, has helped people with an array of chronic conditions — including heart disease, cancer, back pain, and colitis — learn to diminish pain, anxiety and depression through a program that integrates meditation, yoga, and group support.
- Stanford University School of Medicine, where David Spiegel, M.D., professor of psychiatry and behavioral sciences, has led support groups for women with metastatic breast cancer. Combining the sharing of powerful and painful feelings about illness and death with self-hypnosis and guided imagery, Spiegel's group members not only felt better about themselves, but lived an average of 18 months longer than patients who did not participate.

These results are gaining respect and interest among health care professionals and the public, and, accordingly, they are generating the need for educational programs about this complex, evolving field.

Mind-body health is an approach to well-being that sees the mind — our thoughts, emotions and attitudes — as having a central impact on the body's health. Mind-body health techniques include a variety of treatments such as meditation, relaxation training, exercise, biofeedback, social support groups, hypnosis, psychotherapy and stress management — methods that enlist the mind in improving emotional well-being and physical health.

A basic principle of mind-body health is that it is important to treat the whole person. This tenet includes the belief that treatment of emotional distress should be an essential complement to standard medical care. In other words, we are physical beings, but we are also mental, emotional and spiritual beings. We live within our body, but we also live within a family, society, ethnic group and work force — and all of these are factors in our health status.

A second basic principle of mind-body health is that people should be active participants in their own health care and may be able to prevent disease or shorten its course by taking steps to manage their own psychological and physiological states. Studies have shown that active, assertive patients fare better medically than more passive ones. A patient's relationship with a physician should be one of partnership — this gives a person a sense of being in control of the treatment, which can be therapeutic in and of itself.

The mind-body health perspective recognizes that many factors are at work in health and illness; it does not hold that people can heal themselves simply through the power of positive thinking. However, there is increasing evidence to support the contention that thoughts, emotions and attitudes do affect physical health and that mind-body approaches lessen the severity and frequency of medical symptoms. Also, mind-body approaches play a preventive role by strengthening the body's immune system. These methods, learned, understood and applied within the context of comprehensive conventional medicine, serve as complements to standard medical care.

A GROWING FIELD ENGENDERS STRONG PUBLIC INTEREST

The field of mind-body health has received unprecedented attention in recent years. Since one dramatic day in 1974 when a study at the University of Rochester School of Medicine found that the brain and the immune system are connected and able to influence each other's functioning, a steady, increasing stream of studies on the mind's influence on the body has been completed in three areas:

- physiological research, which investigates the biological and biochemical connections among the body's systems;
- epidemiological research, which shows connections between certain psychological factors and certain illnesses in the population at large; and
- clinical research, which tests the effectiveness of mind-body approaches in preventing, alleviating, or treating specific diseases.

Taken together, this research has begun to show a cohesive picture, one that has prompted a highly visible spate of mind-body health activity in the past five years:

- The National Institutes of Health established an Office of Alternative Medicine in 1992 to support research outside the medical mainstream. Prior to this landmark event, federal funding had rarely been used to study psychological interventions and mind-body techniques.
- *The New England Journal of Medicine* published a national survey reporting that one out of three Americans used at least one unconventional therapy in 1990. The survey concluded that "unconventional medicine has an enormous presence in the U.S. health care system."
- *Healing and the Mind With Bill Moyers*, a five part public television series on mind-body health topics, aired to wide public and critical

acclaim; and Bill Moyers' companion book of the same title became a national bestseller.

The result of this activity has been a dramatic increase in the public's interest in the field of mind-body health — an interest replete with the quest for information and answers that typically surrounds emerging fields.

Public interest in mind-body health has been further spurred by the current national debate on how to overhaul and put the "human touch" back into the country's health care system. In 1991, annual medical costs in the U.S. were more than $750 billion, more than twelve percent of our gross national product, while Japan, America's major economic rival spends six percent of its gross national product. Yet, the United States ranks lower than most of these nations on most major indicators of national health, including infant mortality. Mind-body health techniques are inexpensive and do not involve highly technical interventions. With its lower cost, and more accessible, low-technology approach, mind-body health is perceived by many as offering an important means of reducing escalating health costs while creating a heightened sense of well-being, increased sense of control over life, enhanced health, more rapid recovery, and a lessening of suffering for the chronically ill.

In all, citizens in communities across the country are expressing a curiosity about how healing is related to the mind. Does stress make people susceptible to illness? Is anxiety detrimental to the immune system that defends against disease? Does depression raise vulnerability to colds, flu, even heart attacks? Does patient optimism or pessimism affect health status? As research findings to these compelling questions become available, educational programs for the public become an imperative.

A LEADERSHIP OPPORTUNITY
FOR COMMUNITY COLLEGES:
CREATING A CLIMATE FOR MIND-BODY HEALTH STUDIES

> *"The term `community' should be defined ... as a climate to be created. The building of community, in its broadest and best sense, encompasses a concern for the whole, for integration and collaboration, for openness and integrity, for inclusiveness and self-renewal."*
>
> ***A Report of the Commission on the Future***
> ***of Community Colleges, 1988***

Community colleges — the people's colleges — have traditionally responded in timely, innovative ways to the educational needs of the citizens they serve. Growth in public awareness of the possibilities that mind-body health presents, when juxtaposed with a striking lack of public information and education about the field and its evolving knowledge-base, offers the community college the kind of challenge it is accustomed to meeting. Through the range of ways in which it delivers education — academic disciplines, community services, and continuing education — community colleges can help the members of their respective communities understand what mind-body health is, how it can complement traditional medicine, the options it offers them, how to apply its various approaches to their lives, and where applicable, how to become a practitioner of its various techniques.

Community colleges are well-positioned to assume leadership roles in this new educational realm by providing health care professionals and the general public with a responsive environment in which the study of mind-body health — its history, its underpinning philosophy, and its applications — can be pursued.

SUGGESTIONS FOR COMMUNITY COLLEGE LEADERS

In order to further opportunities for the study of mind-body health at community colleges, the AACC/Fetzer Institute Roundtable offers the following suggestions:

Community college leaders are encouraged to:

1. Create a campus climate that is receptive to the legitimate exploration of ideas, topics and applications in the evolving field of mind-body health; one that views health in terms that are free of both charlatanism and unyielding orthodoxy.

2. Examine their college mission statements to determine where the study of mind-body health coincides with the college's current purposes. For example, many colleges will find that a commitment to "educating the whole person" is already a part of their mission. As well, many colleges will find that the study of mind-body health has already found a place within their curriculum.

3. Appoint a mind-body health advisory group, comprised of faculty, students, administrators, and community leaders, to determine the college's and the community's level of interest in mind-body health, and where fitting, recommend avenues for integrating the study of mind-body health into the college's educational offerings.

4. Provide opportunities for faculty and students already interested in mind-body health to pursue these interests.

5. Increase awareness and understanding among faculty, administrators, students and community members of this new, evolving area of study and its ramifications for health, healing and overall well-being.

The American Association of Community Colleges (AACC), Fetzer Institute and other interested groups are encouraged to:

1. Work to clarify the language that surrounds the field of mind-body health, and in so doing, bring coherence to the way in which both health care professionals and the public understand the distinctions between such terms as "mind-body health," "wellness," "holistic medicine," and "complementary medicine."

2. Develop a range of mind-body health educational resources such as course outlines, sample syllabi, study guides, reading lists, videos, public information guides and suggested formats for classroom and continuing education/community service programs.

3. Conduct a set of pilot programs reflective of a range of approaches to the study of mind-body health (i.e. credit and non-credit courses, seminars and study groups, and the infusion of mind-body health precepts into existing courses and programs), and broadly distribute case studies of these programs to all community colleges.

Part IV

ROUNDTABLE
BACKGROUND PAPERS

- What is Mind/Body Medicine?
  by Daniel Goleman, Ph.D. and Joel Gurin

- Mind-Body Health: The Qualities of a
  New Health Care Model
  by James S. Gordon, M.D.

- A Survey of Mind-Body Health Studies at
  Community Colleges
  by Katherine Bracey Lorenzo, Ph.D.

WHAT IS MIND/BODY MEDICINE?

BY DANIEL GOLEMAN, PH.D. AND JOEL GURIN

- At the University of Massachusetts Medical Center, 30 patients with diverse medical conditions — including heart disease, cancer, diabetes, chronic back pain, and colitis — sit meditating with eyes closed, focusing in utter stillness on the feeling of their breath moving in and out of their bodies. Most people who make this simple practice a part of their daily routine report a lessening of their distress and even relief from many medical symptoms.

- At the Ohio State University College of Medicine, second year students undergoing the stress of final exams are taught a relaxation technique. Blood tests of immune function show that the stress of exams weakens the student's resistance to viruses. But those who practice the relaxation method most diligently show the least impairment of resistance.

- At a hospital in Cleveland, children with chronic, intractable pain from cancer are being taught to escape it by visualizing themselves in a relaxed, happy place.

Such studies are producing an ever-growing body of evidence that portends a sea change in the way health-care professionals and patients are viewing the role of the mind in the treatment of illness. Relaxation, hypnosis, and other mind/body approaches have been used in Western medicine for decades, even centuries, and very possibly for millennia by traditional healers. Two things are different today. First the use of these approaches is becoming more widespread and they are gaining more respect and interest from researchers in major medical institutions. And second, evidence is mounting that mind/body techniques may not only improve the quality of life — particularly for someone dealing with a serious illness — but actually affect the course of the disease itself.

The most compelling study to date was done at Stanford University by David Spiegel, a psychiatrist who never anticipated that his work would show that the mind has an impact on physical health. In the mid-1970s, Spiegel had led support groups for women being treated for advanced breast cancer that had spread throughout the body — a pattern that carries the grimmest of prognoses. His intent

Daniel Goleman writes for The New York Times *on health and human behavior. Joel Gurin is Science Editor of* Consumer Reports.

was to show that women placed at random into these groups, which allowed them to talk over their day-to-day troubles in a supportive setting would suffer less from the emotional distress that accompanies cancer than other women in the same medical situation. The experiment was a success; the data soon showed that the groups did improve the women's quality of life.

The surprise came a decade later, when Spiegel went back to the women's records to see how long they had survived after the groups had disbanded. As he recalls, his original intention was to disprove the notion, spread by some popular books in the mid-1980s, that mental and emotional factors could influence the course of cancer. Instead, he was surprised to find that the women in the support groups had survived twice as long as the others. The added months of life — 18 months on average — were more than even cancer medications could have been expected to provide at that point in the women's disease. When Spiegel published these findings in the journal *The Lancet* late in 1989, they stunned the medical community and inspired many treatments. At least half a dozen research teams are now in the process of repeating his study to see if his results can be replicated.

Other scientists, laboring to unravel the physiology of the mind/body connection, have begun to outline plausible ways in which the mind and emotions could affect physical health. They have deepened our understanding of the effects of stress on the body and are accumulating convincing evidence that the immune system, along with other organs and systems in the body, can be influenced by the mind.

Taken together, these research efforts and clinical experiments suggest that the split between mind and body, long taken for granted in Western philosophy, is illusory indeed. The studies are also part of a new synthesis in medical science. They are part of *mind/body medicine*: an approach that sees the mind — our thoughts and emotions — as having a central impact on the body's health.

For patients, this new synthesis has a very practical significance. It means that by paying attention to and exerting some control over emotional and mental states — your worries, hostility, habitual reactions, pessimism, and depression — you may help yourself stay healthy or recover more rapidly from being sick.

From the perspective of doctors, nurses, and other health-care professionals, this new way of seeing things suggests there is much to be gained if they go beyond attending to physical disease and attend as well to the overall experience of illness — the way the disease affects a patient's spirits and the emotional reactions it calls forth.

In short, one basic tenet of mind/body medicine is that it is best to treat the whole person: Treating emotional distress should be an essential complement to standard medical care. Another tenet is that people can be active participants in their own health care and may be able to prevent disease or shorten its course by taking steps to manage their own psychological states.

Of course, these principles must be tempered with a relativistic view of the many other factors at work in health and illness. No one is promising that people can cure themselves of disease just by thinking happy thoughts. That simplistic idea ignores the complexities of biology and the wired-in destiny of our genes. Worse, it can leave people feeling guilty about being sick at all. That is not the message of mind/body medicine.

But the evidence is growing stronger that states of mind can affect physical health. And while that effect may not be as dramatic as, say, the power of penicillin to fight a strep throat, it can be meaningful nonetheless. Mind/body approaches can certainly reduce the severity and frequency of medical symptoms. For example they can make chronic headaches less frequent, reduce the nausea that accompanies chemotherapy, speed recovery from surgery, and help people with arthritis feel less restricted by their pain. Moreover, the same approaches may help strengthen the body's resistance to disease.

THE QUIET BEGINNINGS

The research that laid the basic scientific foundation for modern mind/body medicine began with an accidental discovery that attracted little attention at first. That discovery was made one day in 1974, in a laboratory at the University of Rochester School of Medicine and Dentistry. It led to research that would redraw biology's map of the body.

On that day, psychologist Robert Ader analyzed data from an experiment showing that the immune systems of white rats had learned a specific conditioned reaction. The results were startling because the prevailing wisdom held that the immune system should not have been capable of learning anything. Learning was something done only by the brain and central nervous system — certainly not by the immune system, the body's disease fighting network of cells.

The discovery was serendipitous. Ader had been conducting a classic Pavlovian conditioning experiment, trying to teach the rats to respond with aversion to saccharin-flavored water. His study had a simple design. The rats were given a drink of saccharin-laced water and then received an injection of the drug cyclophosphamide, which Ader gave them to produce nausea. One shot should have been enough to condition them to associate saccharin water with nausea and avoid it.

But there was a problem. For some reason, many of the rats — though young and healthy — were getting sick and dying. Looking into the problem, Ader realized that the drug he was using to nauseate the rats also suppressed their immune systems. In particular, it lowered the number of T-cells, immune system cells that fight viruses and infections as they circulate through the body.

It seemed to Ader that giving the rats the saccharin water alone, without the immunosuppressive medication, was decreasing the number of T-cells in the rats' bloodstreams. Classical conditioning had triggered a learned association between the taste of saccharin and the suppression of T-cells, so that later — when the rats tasted the flavored water alone — their immune systems reacted as though they were exposed to the drug itself. And that, in turn, made them more susceptible to disease.

But that just should not have happened, according to what was then the best scientific understanding of how the brain and immune system function. Immune system cells travel the entire body, contacting virtually every other cell. Those cells they recognize, they leave alone; those they do not recognize, they attack — defending the body against tumors and virus-infected cells.

Until Ader's experiment, anatomists, physicians, and biologists all believed that the brain and the immune system were separate entities, neither one able to influence the functioning of the other. They were not aware of any pathway that connected the brain centers monitoring what the rats tasted with the areas of bone marrow that manufacture T-cells.

Ader himself could not quite believe his findings. To test the possibility of a connection, he teamed up with Nicholas Cohen, an immunologist at Rochester. In an elegant series of studies, they demonstrated that aspects of the immune system can, in fact, be conditioned, just as Pavlov had shown that dogs can be conditioned to salivate at the sound of a bell after food had been paired with sound.

Ader's experiments have now been repeated successfully, and his discovery has opened the way to identifying the links between the immune system and the central nervous system. As a result, science is finding that there are many physiological connections between these two systems. These findings have generated the field of medical science know as psychoneuroimmunology, or PNI: *psycho* for mind, *neuro* for neuroendocrine system (the nervous and hormonal systems), and immunology for the immune system.

While no one is quite yet sure just how the connections among these areas function, few medical researchers now doubt that such connections exist. Ader likes to quote a basic immunology textbook, published in 1991, that teaches that research studies in PNI "now confirm the long standing belief that the immune system does not function completely autonomously." In the last decade, he says, the reaction of the scientific community to PNI "has gone from, 'It's impossible,' to, 'We knew it all along.'"

An explosion of interest in PNI has brought about some renewed research on a whole range of physiological mechanisms, some of them known for decades, by which the mind and emotions may affect physical well-being. As scientists learn more about the hormones and neurotransmitters that brain cells use to communicate with each other and with the rest of the body, they are developing a deeper understanding of the stress response. They are learning more precisely how the physiological changes that occur under stress — or with emotional distress — may, for example, raise the risk of heart disease, make diabetes more difficult to control, or make it harder for some women to conceive.

Research is now revealing a range of likely avenues through which our mental states may influence our health. Although it will take years of work to piece together the precise biological mechanisms involved, the research done so far provides the beginnings of a sound scientific basis for mind/body medicine.

THREE LINES OF EVIDENCE

The scientific evidence for the mind's influence on the body now comes from three converging areas of research:

- Physiological research, which investigates the biological and biochemical connections between the brain and the body's systems.
- Epidemiological research, which shows correlations between certain psychological factors and certain illnesses in the population at large.
- Clinical research which tests the effectiveness of mind/body approaches in preventing, alleviating, or treating specific diseases.

Each of these areas, taken alone, is incomplete; each has produced promising findings, but also raised unanswered questions. Taken together, however, the different kinds of research in mind/body medicine are beginning to show a coherent picture — like a jigsaw puzzle that still has many pieces missing, but that is starting to form a recognizable image.

Physiological research in mind/body medicine dates back to Walter B. Cannon, who discovered the "fight-or-flight response" to stress during World War I. But the modern study of the mind/body physiology began in the 1940s, when the pioneer researcher Hans Selye investigated the physical effects of psychological stress. This avenue of investigation was a precursor of current physiological research, which ranges from studying the intricacies of PNI to examining the ways in which emotions like anger may lead to biological changes that raise heart attack risk.

The key question for physiological researchers is whether the biological changes that stem from psychological factors actually make a difference to health. For example, even if stress or depression does lower the effectiveness of the immune system, is the drop great enough to increase the risk of illness? In addition, because many physiological studies are done on experimental animals, their relevance may be uncertain.

Epidemiological studies in this field look for relationships between psychosocial factors and patterns of illness in large populations. They date back to the early 1960s, when a study done for the U.S. Navy showed that men who had gone through serious life change — a divorce, move, job loss, or the like — had an increased chance of becoming seriously ill within the months following the upsets. A more recent, and very significant, series of studies covering thousands of people has shown that men and women with few social ties are significantly more likely to become ill and die than people with a rich network of family, friends, and other social involvements.

The provocative findings of studies like these often suggest avenues for both physiological and clinical research. For instance, some researchers are now trying to unravel the reasons why upsetting experiences may be associated with illness and why strong social networks are linked to better health.

Clinical research provides the third major line of evidence, one that is now getting increased attention. David Spiegel's work with support groups for women with breast cancer is a paradigm of the new research in this area. The main shortcomings here are that such studies, while promising, must be seen as preliminary until they can be repeated by other, independent scientific investigators. And even then, without carefully designed follow-up studies of the people treated, it is by no means clear how and why such interventions may work. For instance, support groups for patients may work because they encourage patients to comply better with what their physicians tell them to do, or because the emotional changes the groups produce help boost immunity directly — or for both reasons.

The issues become even more complex when social support and relaxation training are combined with changes in diet and exercise, as they were in one of the most impressive clinical studies in this field. Internist Dean Ornish, director of the Preventative Medicine Research Institute at the University of California, San Francisco, conducted a study with patients who had severe coronary heart disease.

He placed them in groups and led them through several significant life-style changes, combining mind/body approaches with a very low-fat diet (one in which fat accounted for less than ten percent of total calories). After one year in the groups, patients showed actual reversal of their severe atherosclerosis, something that had never previously been accomplished without the use of medication. Ornish's further research is showing that, in general, an even greater degree of reversal occurs in people who stay on the program over several years.

But the success of Ornish's patients cannot be attributed to any single, isolated part of the program, even though each part of the program was correlated independently with reversal of heart disease. The patients made full use of several mind/body approaches: They met weekly to share their life-styles to lead less stressful, more fulfilling lives; and they practiced yoga and meditation. They also began to exercise several hours a week — a change that, in itself, can have significant effects on mood and mind.

A large number of new clinical studies are now under way at leading U.S. medical institutions to measure the effects of mind/body techniques and to explore the physiological basis for those effects. Here are just a few examples of those studies:

- At Harvard Medical School, a series of ongoing studies suggests that a simple technique for eliciting the body's "relaxation response" can help patients with diseases ranging from hypertension to migraine headaches to irritable bowel syndrome.

- At Duke University, men and women with cardiovascular disease participate in groups that help them control their feelings of hostility and anger. (Earlier studies at Duke and elsewhere had shown that hostility is a risk factor for heart disease). The researchers will follow the patients over time to see whether these emotional changes directly help their hearts.

- At the University of California, Los Angeles, a prospective study has been designed to follow up on David Spiegel's groundbreaking findings. Support groups for cancer patients at UCLA have already been found to strengthen key elements of the immune system. These patients are now being studied to see whether the immunological changes are correlated with better clinical results, such as longer survival.

- At the University of Miami, the focus is on AIDS. There, in a comprehensive stress management program, men with HIV infection meet on Monday and Thursday nights to talk over the stresses of the week, to practice relaxation methods, and to help each other find ways to improve how they handle the range of life's demands. Again, early results are promising: heightened emotional resilience, positive effects on the immune system, and a delay in the onset of the more serious physical symptoms that signal AIDS.

Mind/body medicine is still far from being an exact science, and many perplexing questions remain. But the areas of uncertainty are no greater than one would expect in a complex, evolving field. And the volume of the well-designed research now under way or just beginning attests to the scientific excitement the field has generated in a fairly short period of time.

For most people, the question is not whether mind/body medicine is a legitimate field for research (it is) or whether its potential has been fully defined and proven (not yet). The immediate, practical question is whether mind/body medicine as it now stands can be of value to people dealing with a range of serious illnesses and to healthy people who want to stay that way.

We believe that it can. Although mind/body medicine is still evolving, enough is now known to make it worth trying in a number of situations. It may do a great deal to improve patient's quality of life, and possibly to improve their physical health with very little risk.

A key reason is that mind/body medicine is not so much an "alternative" approach as a complementary one. It is perfectly compatible with standard medical treatment and can be a powerful way of augmenting it, not challenging or replacing it. In fact, the mind/body approach harkens back to some of the best traditions of Western medicine — although some of those traditions have been ignored in the expanding, high-tech era of modern health care.

BEYOND THE PLACEBO

Long before research in PNI began, the mind's power to affect the body was well known in medicine. In the centuries before antibiotics and other "miracle drugs," caring physicians hoped that a reassuring bedside manner would mobilize hidden resources within their patients to fight their illness, and they consciously used the power of the mind to help heal the body. This approach was essential in the days when physicians had relatively few effective medications or procedures to offer; indeed, a motto of medicine until a century ago was, "Comfort always, heal seldom."

But the tradition drew on a deeper wisdom that can be traced back to Hippocrates: The understanding that the physician's manner is as potent as many a medicine. For centuries, wise doctors tried to capitalize upon the *placebo effect*, the power for healing that can stem simply from a patient's belief that a treatment will be effective.

Offering patients hope and reassurances may seem quaint in a day when finally, the doctor's bag contains medications that are truly effective and the tools of medicine daily grows more technologically dazzling. Yet the power of the placebo is still very real. In fact, it is implicitly acknowledged by every major medical journal in the world, as well as the U.S. Food and Drug Administration. The scientific method now requires that every new drug must be tested against a placebo, a dummy medication given to patients as if it was a real drug.

The optimum study is prospective, randomized, and double blind. Patients are divided at random into two groups: One receives the real drug, the other receives a look alike placebo, and neither the patient nor the physician knows which is which (a necessary precaution because that knowledge itself could affect the outcome). If the placebo effect were not a powerful one — powerful enough to derail an otherwise careful medical experiment — such elaborate precautions would be unnecessary.

The placebo effect has long puzzled medical researchers, who were at a loss to explain it but unable to dismiss it. Study after study showed that, for virtually any disease, a substantial portion of the symptoms — roughly one-third, by most estimates — would improve when patients were given a placebo treatment with no pharmacological activity. Patients simply believes that the treatment would help the, and somehow, it did.

Although some medical researchers may think of the placebo effect as the experimental "static" than can interfere with an otherwise clean study, it is a striking demonstration of the mind's effect on health. In many ways, mind/body medicine is an attempt to harness the same forces that are behind the placebo effect, but in ways that enable patients to become active partners with their physicians in helping to heal themselves.

REHUMANIZING MEDICINE

Unfortunately, the development of modern medicine has made that kind of partnership more difficult to achieve. Over the last few decades, medicine has become more centered on high technology, physicians have become more specialized into narrow niches, and economics has forced doctors to spend less time with each patient. Physicians are not reimbursed as well for talking and listening to their patients as they are for performing tests and administering treatments. Although many physicians and nurses still offer their patients sensitive care, too many lack both the time and the training to help patients deal with their anxieties and other emotions — even though a patients emotional state can be closely related to his or her physical health and can influence the course of treatment and recovery.

There is now a growing movement within medical schools and medical specialty organizations to improve the doctor/patient relationship. That movement has been fueled largely by evidence that many people find their physicians insensitive to their needs: Surveys show considerable dissatisfaction with conventional medical care, and the growing interest in "alternative" practices like chiropractic, acupuncture, and homeopathy certainly reflects it. There is also increasing evidence showing that good communication between doctor and patient can have a direct, beneficial effect on physical health.

Because the doctor/patient relationship has long been considered a major part of medical care, many physicians should welcome this return to traditional values. But effective, caring communication is only part of mind/body medicine, although an important part. Mind/body medicine also includes a number of specific self-help techniques — such as relaxation training, meditation, hypnosis, and biofeedback — that physicians may be unfamiliar with and may view with suspicion. In general, these approaches are barely covered in medical school, if they're mentioned at all.

Physicians are also likely to be unaware of the research that has made mind/body medicine a more credible field within the last decade. Older physicians may have received some exposure to "psychosomatic" medicine during their training. But many psychosomatic theories of disease — such as the notion that specific personality types predispose people to different kinds of illness — have not held up over time. Younger physicians may have learned something about the concepts of psychoneuroimmunology, but only if they were recent medical school graduates — and only if they had the interest to pursue these concepts.

Even physicians who follow the medical literature faithfully could have missed the development of mind/body medicine. Much of the research in this field has been published in journals of psychiatry or psychology or in journals that cover individual medical specialties. Relatively few research papers have been published in the most widely read journals, such as *The Lancet* and *The New England Journal of Medicine*, although some recent key papers in those journals have brought mind/body medicine to more general attention. As the quality of mind/body research continues to improve — and it has improved dramatically in the last few years — the number of reports in major mainstream journals should also increase.

Ultimately, many physicians may be hesitant to use mind/body approaches for a fundamental reason: The new field of mind/body medicine is still in search of a comprehensive, unifying theory. Psychoneuroimmunology, which comes closest, is still incomplete from a scientific point of view. The working hypothesis for much PNI research is that psychological distress can suppress the immune system; that this effect can be great enough to increase the risk of physical illness; and that people who learn relaxation, stress management, or other mind/body approaches can increase their immunological resistance to disease. But although that hypothesis is consistent with a growing body of evidence, it is still far from proven.

THE CERTAIN BELIEFS

If research in PNI were the only justification for using mind/body approaches it would certainly be premature to use them widely. But because there is strong evidence supporting their use, we believe that physicians, psychologists, and other health-care professionals should be using these approaches more extensively than they are doing now, for several reasons:

- Many of the links between mind and body have little or nothing to do with the immune system. Psychological stress can also affect the endocrine (hormonal) system and the circulatory system in ways that can be useful in managing a number of illnesses related to those systems, from migraine headaches to diabetes.

- There is abundant evidence that psychological factors affect the way people experience medical symptoms, even when the mind does not affect the underlying disease process. Two people with chronic pain, for example, may have precisely the same underlying physical problem and yet, for psychological reasons, one may function reasonably well while the other is incapacitated. The same can be said of people with arthritis or irritable bowel syndrome. In some cases, psychological problems can lead to debilitating physical symptoms in people who have no diagnosable medical illness at all. Psychotherapy, stress management, and other mind/body approaches can do a great deal to help those people reduce their symptoms — and their medical bills.

- It is now indisputable that mind/body approaches can greatly improve the quality of life for people with physical illnesses. This is especially clear for people with cancer, a terrifying disease and one whose primary treatments, radiation and chemotherapy, have extremely unpleasant side effects. Relaxation methods, hypnosis, psychotherapy, and support groups like David Spiegel's have all been shown to help cancer patients deal effectively with their fears and anxieties about the disease and the treatments they must take. Even if these mind/body approaches did not extend the life of a single cancer patient, their emotional benefits would make them a valuable part of every cancer patient's care.

• Finally, the physical and emotional risks of mind/body techniques are virtually non-existent. Even if some of their benefits are still hypothetical, no one is likely to be harmed by giving these approaches a try — as long as they're not used in place of conventional medicine.

WHAT DOES IT COST?

Mind/body approaches are generally inexpensive; some are even free. It costs next to nothing, for example, to learn the "relaxation response" — a basic method of meditation that is now used to treat a range of physical problems. Participation in groups that teach other forms of meditation, such as "mindfulness" meditation, generally costs little or nothing. If you want to use relaxation or meditation to help you deal with a medical problem, however, you should discuss your specific program with your doctor, at the cost of a medical consultation.

Self-help groups for people with different medical problems offer social support, now recognized as a major psychological aid — and these too, cost little or nothing to join. Some groups offer specific education in dealing with a disease, which can have both practical value and the psychological value of helping you feel a greater sense of control. A model for this approach, the Arthritis Self-Help Course, is now offered at hundreds of locations by the Arthritis Foundation, at an average cost of about $20.

Hospital-based stress management courses can be considerably more expensive. One well-respected program costs just over $500 for eight group sessions plus two individual sessions. Other programs may cost twice as much, or more.

At the high end of the scale are the individualized approaches: hypnosis, biofeedback, and psychotherapy. Costs for these treatments can range from around $50 a session to over $100. Biofeedback and hypnosis, however, are designed to help you learn to regulate your mind and your body on your own; you will need only a limited number of sessions with a professional. And many physical problems that can be helped with psychotherapy require only a few months or less of weekly sessions.

Anyone thinking of trying a fee-based approach will naturally want to know how much of the cost is covered by medical insurance. There is no clear answer. In fact, the level of insurance reimbursement can vary from nearly complete to nothing at all. It depends on such factors as the policies of the insurance carrier, the nature of the mind/body approach, the setting in which the treatment is given (such as a hospital or a private office), and the reason for the treatment. For example, someone who learns biofeedback to help control Raynaud's disease — a circulatory problem for which biofeedback is a well-recognized treatment — will be more likely to be reimbursed than someone who enters psychotherapy to deal with more general emotional problems (even though these problems may affect physical health).

Overall, mind/body approaches are generally not reimbursed at the same rate as conventional medical treatments. Most insurance companies, for instance, pay only 50 percent of the cost of psychotherapy as opposed to 80 percent for other procedures). In addition, they set low limits for the allowable cost per session and for the total amount that will be reimbursed over the life of the policy.

Such limits are unfortunate, because there is increasing evidence that psychological interventions can not only alleviate suffering but also reduce the overall cost of treatment. A number of studies have shown that people with medical problems who undergo psychotherapy lower their medical bills enough to pay for their therapy, and more. Similarly, certain kinds of psychological preparation for surgery can speed a patient's recovery enough to save many dollars in hospital costs — $1,000 or more, according to studies of some procedures. Although these studies are not definitive, the evidence so far suggests that the mind/body approaches may be highly cost-effective.

On top of that, no one has even begun to estimate the potential savings, both in illness and in dollars, of using mind/body approaches to prevent disease as well as treat it. Preventive care in general has gotten short shrift from our medical institutions and third-party payers, which largely follow a disease management model, one that focuses on the treatment of symptoms and diseases only after they emerge. As a society, however, we are being forced to confront the economic costs of slighting disease prevention. In 1992, health-care costs in the United States exceeded $800 billion. By the year 2000, at the present rate of increase, that figure would more than double, and make up roughly 20 percent of the projected gross national product.

Something has to change. And one reasonable alternative, among many, is to emphasize disease prevention by encouraging a healthy life-style — including mind/body methods — particularly for groups of people at risk for specific diseases. To the degree that emotional turmoil and stress speed the disease process, mind/body interventions might well save money as well as protect health. Although these benefits are not yet proven, the possibility is already leading forward-looking insurance companies, health-care organizations, and corporations to examine mind/body methods as one way to decrease the cost of medical care.

THE BOTTOM LINE

Mind/body medicine includes a variety of treatments and approaches, ranging from meditation and relaxation to social support groups, that are designed to enlist the mind in improving well-being and physical health. A growing body of research now supports the use of these techniques. Nevertheless, they are probably being used by only a fraction of the people who could benefit from them.

Although many questions about mind/body medicine remain to be answered, we believe mind/body approaches can and should become much more widely used as a regular part of medical care, for several reasons:

- Mind/body approaches have shown great potential for improving the quality of life and reducing the pain and difficulty of symptoms for people with various chronic diseases.
- They may help control or reverse certain underlying disease processes.
- By reducing the effects of stress, they may help to prevent disease from developing.
- The physical and emotional risk of using these techniques is minimal while their potential benefit is high.
- The economic cost of most mind/body approaches is low; many can be taught by paraprofessionals and involve no high-tech interventions.
- These techniques can easily be applied in the context of conventional medicine, rather than standing in opposition to it. They can and should be used along with standard medical care.

Despite encouraging trends, both physicians and insurance companies are lagging behind the needs of ordinary patients. More and more people are looking for medical care that takes into account their thoughts and emotions as well as their overt medical problems — in short, mind/body medicine. Informed consumers who want to try a mind/body approach often want answers to a number of questions that their doctors may not be able to help them with: What actually works? What is known about these methods and their strengths and limitations? And how do you find a reliable practitioner?

Our book, *Mind/Body Medicine*, is designed to answer such crucial questions, as fully as current scientific knowledge allows — as do the other publications listed in this monograph's resources section beginning on page 39.

MIND-BODY HEALTH: THE QUALITIES OF A NEW HEALTH CARE MODEL

BY JAMES S. GORDON

The following is a summary of remarks presented by Dr. Gordon at the AACC/Fetzer Institute Mind-Body Health Community College Roundtable, March 14-15, 1995, Kalamazoo, Michigan.

The characteristics of mind-body health comprise the heart of what health care should be about, and will be about, in my opinion. Today we are seeing a profound shift away from the current, physician-dominated, biomedical model of what illness care is about, to a new collaborative model of what health care is about. Health care in the United States is slowly moving in a progressive direction to include aspects of mind-body health that many of us have been trying to bring into higher education curricula. My prediction is that in twenty years this expanded view of health care will become standard.

Microbiologist Rene Dubos pointed this out in 1959 in his book, *Mirage of Health*. He suggested that we are beginning to come to the end of the biomedical era. We have made enormous advances with biomedicine. We have wonderful surgical and pharmacological techniques. Although we can still appreciate the power of this biomedical approach in curing infections and treating acute illnesses, in the years since the publication of *Mirage of Health*, we have begun to see how difficult it is to use these methods to treat a variety of chronic and stress-related illnesses. We have become painfully aware of the side effects and overuse of once promising therapies.

During the last two decades both patients and physicians have become increasingly impatient with the kind of care that they have been receiving and offering. They feel a lack of participation and partnership. According to polls taken by Gallup and the American Medical Association itself, there is a sense of alienation on both sides.

James S. Gordon, M.D., is a clinical professor in the Departments of Psychiatry and Family Medicine at Georgetown University School of Medicine, and Director of The Center for Mind-Body Medicine in Washington, D.C.

During this time, as well, the world has become smaller and more intimate. We have become aware of the healing traditions of other cultures, and of approaches that have been ignored or scorned within our own culture. And finally, we have become acutely sensitive to the huge financial drain that our medical system is putting on our government and all of us. Health care required four percent of the Gross National Product when Dubos was writing in the 1950's. Now, it is almost fifteen percent.

Taken together, these forces have set the stage for a new model of health care which I will characterize below. As educators, we should recognize that education is fundamental to the new model of health care. It is not simply a matter of teaching a new course, or presenting new information. The basis of health care in the future is going to be health education.

The semantics involved in labeling the new model are tangled. Sometimes we call it *mind-body medicine* to emphasize the kind of complete interpenetration of mind and body — the effects of the mind on the body and the effects of the body on the mind — both of which were largely neglected, except in the narrowest biochemical sense, by modern medicine. Sometimes we call it *holistic medicine*. In many ways, that is a better term. It conveys the notion of a whole person in his or her total environment, and of the whole spectrum of therapeutic possibilities coming together. *Wellness* is also a powerful term, but it does not capture the fact that these are not simply approaches that are useful when you are feeling well, but these are also fundamental treatments for illness. And finally, *alternative* and *complementary*. Alternative is a term of opposition. It connotes everything that doctors did not learn in medical school. It can be everything that is not conventionally practiced in hospitals, or in most clinic settings. Complementary is a slightly more friendly term. It describes bringing together those things that are not practiced conventionally with those that are practiced conventionally.

Each of these terms has its uses, but the bottom line is that we are talking about a comprehensive medicine, one that includes alternative and conventional, one that adopts a humanistic approach, one that is holistic, one that is based on an understanding of the total interpenetration of mind and body. I believe the current semantic entanglement is due to the fact that we are seeking a name for things that should be absolutely obvious. The reason we have to seek a name is only due to the fact that we have lost track of what is fundamental to health care and healing. For the time being, different people will be using different names, and that is fine. But my sense is that in the future, what we are going to be talking about is simply medicine and health care, and that this new model is going to be at the heart of it.

I want to outline seven aspects or qualities of what this new model of health care is all about:

INDIVIDUALS ARE UNIQUE

In the mental health field today, the first question professionals ask is "into what diagnostic category does the patient fit?" and, depending on the diagnostic category, "what drug do we give the patient?" In this way the uniqueness of each individual gets lost in the avalanche of diagnoses and prescriptions. Uniqueness is not solely psychological or sociological. Uniqueness is also deeply biological. For example, I may need 50 milligrams of Vitamin C. You may need 1500 milligrams. We are that different, one to the other. You may need 1500 milligrams of Vitamin C and only two milligrams of thiamine, and I may need the reverse. This notion of biological uniqueness is all but lost in our current medical setting where we have uniform formulas for all patients that eliminate the appreciation for individuality. At the same time, in our society an increasing number of people are appreciating their own individuality. So there is a curious tugging going on between a medical establishment which is moving in the direction of greater standardization, and popular, educational, and self-help movements, which are paying attention to uniqueness.

HOLISTIC

The second aspect of the mind-body perspective is the holistic one. We are not only physical, we are also mental, emotional, and spiritual beings. We're part of a society, a class, an ethnic group, a family, we have a particular occupation — and all of these play into our sense of who we are and our health status. These factors should be understood and explored when dealing with any given human being.

For example, I live and work in Washington, D.C. where one of the major problems my patients have, regardless of the diagnosis, is stress due to an unbearable job. You cannot effectively help somebody deal with a chronic illness and uproot the hold that a chronic illness has taken on that person without dealing with non-physical aspects. I have found that if someone is in a work situation that is intolerable, it is very hard for them to get well. I think our current health care environment errs by seeing cases in solely biological terms, without consideration of psycho-social and spiritual aspects. A helpful therapy is not always found within the same sphere as the problem being addressed. For example, I find the best single therapy for my patients who are suffering from depression or anxiety is physical exercise. This is not a therapy commonly taught in psychiatric programs. Conversely, psychological aspects must be considered when treating every chronic illness.

ACTIVE PARTICIPATION AND PARTNERSHIP

Work within the new mind-body health care model has to be based on a patient-health professional partnership, rather than on a doctor-directed, top/down flow. Essential to the new model's approach is a gradual shifting of responsibility from the physician to the patient, so that the physician becomes more of a teacher. People must be active participants in their own health care. When I am teaching medical students, I try to instill in them the notion of having a partnership with patients. I have patients come in to talk to our classes at Georgetown Medical School. The patients teach us continually about their illness, about what the medical system is like for a patient, about their own behavior, and about their own ways of thinking. I believe as educators it is essential that we let people know that they should expect and demand a partnership with their physicians and other health care providers. There is significant research on the negative effects of hopelessness and helplessness, as well as the positive effects of people who have a sense of control. Therefore, the notion of a partnership is itself healing. It is not simply about being democratic; it is fundamental to certain kinds of healing.

PRIMARY CARE AS SELF-CARE

The fourth aspect of the new model concerns each person taking primary responsibility for their own care. There are lots of arguments today concerning primary care: Should the nurse practitioner be the primary care provider? Should the family physician be the primary care provider? I believe we should all be our own primary care providers. That does not mean we are totally responsible for our own care. But primary care is what everybody should be taught. This should be fundamental to everybody's education. I am involved in a program in the Washington, D.C. public high schools where we are trying to teach students how to take care of themselves. This should be done in grade school, again in high school, and certainly at the college level. Yet, it's virtually never done. This is fundamental to learning how to live. And it is not only fundamental to being in good health physically, it is a fundamental tool for helping people to be fully human. Because in order to take care of yourself, you have to understand yourself.

I have my medical students keep a diary, try meditation, pay strict attention to what they eat, and do a significant amount of physical exercise. These are all course requirements. How can you work with other people if you do not have a sense of what is going on with you? It is not a part of any medical school's formal curriculum, and yet it should be part of everybody's curriculum. Learning to take care of one's self is a deep educational tool. Becoming sensitive to what is happening in your body and in your life fundamentally changes the way you view the world, from someone who simply is looking for a doctor's expertise, to someone who realizes that he or she can become their own expert care.

UNDERSTANDING THE WORLD'S HEALING SYSTEMS

The fifth quality — and this is very important in an educational institution — is an understanding and perspective on our society's particular ways of healing. What is our Western biomedicine? Where does it come from? What are its strengths and limitations? How does it fit into the larger scheme of all of the world's healing systems? This understanding should be part of every health curriculum because the assumption, up until very recently, has been that we in the West have all the answers. We have discovered, in the last twenty years or so, that this is not the case. Not only do we not have all the answers, but there are other traditions that have answers to problems we are unable solve. And, of course, we have answers to problems they cannot solve.

No amount of Ayurvedic medicine (which has origins in India) or Chinese medicine is going to help you if you have been hit in a severe automobile accident. Conversely, our Western medicine is not very good if you have rheumatoid arthritis. It will relieve the symptoms, but also cause a great many other problems. In an academic setting, it seems very appropriate to teach a cross-cultural approach.

IMPORTANCE OF GROUP SUPPORT

The sixth piece of the new model is the importance of group support. Again, this is something that is not taught. Even most people who run groups see group support as helpful, but not as essential to health care. In mental health care, group therapy is considered a nice adjunct, while individual therapy is thought of as the "real thing." Yet groups have a healing power that individual work does not. I have been involved in a professional training program in Washington to teach people how to work with groups of people with chronic illness, and not just via the psychotherapeutic approach. Group psychotherapy is very important, but it's also important to teach mind-body health approaches — relaxation, meditation, nutrition, exercise, bio-feedback — in a group context. It may well be that group experience is the most powerful therapeutic element. Even though the therapy approach being taught to the group may be diet, exercise or meditation, it may well be the group itself that is the most powerful ingredient.

For the purpose of education, it seems crucial to me for people to have some experience of what it is like to be in a group and engaged in both giving and receiving. Giving to somebody else is absolutely crucial in healing. If you are sick you need to receive care from other people. But it is also true that one of the most healing experiences when you are sick is to be able to give to somebody else. Many of the people I work with who are long-term AIDS survivors tell me that they are convinced, even though they have been using many kinds of conventional and alternative therapies, that helping other people is what is keeping them alive.

SPIRITUAL DIMENSION: SELF-DISCOVERY AND MEANING

And finally, the seventh aspect is the spiritual dimension — a dimension of self-discovery and a deeper sense of meaning. Let me be clear: I do not mean spiritual in necessarily a religious sense. Rather, spiritual by serving a larger purpose in the world. For patients it may be spiritual in the sense that illness can be a path of self-discovery and meaning. For health care professionals and therapists, it is spiritual in the sense that healing is a path of service to fellow human beings. The work that health professionals do is basically a spiritual work. The work also, of course, has to do with the body and the mind. But it is a deeply spiritual work. Historically, healing and spiritual work were always united up until several hundred years ago in the West. Today, in many cultures, they are still completely united.

Healing is spiritual in two senses. One is that illness does represent an opportunity to learn. What can we learn from it? My own experience, and that of probably thousands of people with whom I have worked, is that illness has taught them something very powerful. Perhaps it taught them about factors that may have contributed to their illness. Or perhaps it taught them something about themselves as they deal with the illness. Or it has taught them about what has been left undone in their lives. Lawrence LeShan, Ph.D., has written a book on this topic with a wonderful title: *Cancer As A Turning Point.* Basketball star Earvin "Magic" Johnson called his struggle with being HIV-positive a wake-up call. Illness as an opportunity for learning — if nothing else, it redeems you from being utterly miserable.

Health care practitioners and therapists are also engaged in a spiritual enterprise. It is not merely a matter of learning about illness and learning about disease. It is learning about ourselves in the course of being helpful to other people, as practitioners or teachers. And this sense of service, this spirituality, for me anyway, takes the whole enterprise of health care and health education out of the technical and psychological realms. As important as the physical and psychological are, as important as gaining technical expertise and book learning are, seeing this healing work as a way for a kind of spiritual development, puts it in an entirely other dimension where each learning, each interaction, each day has a powerful value to all of us.

There is an opportunity today to create a new, more comprehensive kind of health care system. The climate is right for a synthesis of approaches that is all-encompassing. No one system has all the answers — whether its conventional Western medicine, Chinese medicine or Indian medicine. We need to take what is useful from the traditions of different healing systems and combine them. We have before us a wonderful opportunity to help people in new ways.

A SURVEY OF MIND-BODY HEALTH STUDIES AT COMMUNITY COLLEGES

BY KATHERINE BRACEY LORENZO

In Fall, 1994, the American Association of Community Colleges and the Fetzer Institute embarked upon a joint initiative to explore if and how the nation's community colleges might respond with information and education on mind-body health to increasing public interest in this area. As a first step it was decided to conduct a state-of-the-art survey. The purpose of this survey was to determine what is currently taking place in regards to the study of mind-body health on community college campuses across the country. The survey results then served as background information for participants in the Mind-Body Health Community College Roundtable jointly conducted March 14-15, 1995 by the American Association of Community Colleges and the Fetzer Institute.

The survey materials were developed in late 1994 and mailed to the leadership of approximately 2,000 community college campuses in this country and Canada, both public and private. Each set of survey materials included a letter of introduction and explanation addressed to the institution's chief executive officer, along with two survey forms. . . one to be completed by the academic dean, the other to be completed by the dean of continuing education or community services.

Because of our interest in assessing the status of mind-body health studies only, a distinction was made within the survey forms between mind-body health and what is commonly know as *wellness*. The following definitions were provided for clarification:

Wellness: Strategies designed to reduce health risk and enhance quality of life through wise lifestyle choices. Examples of wellness programs or classes include blood pressure and cholesterol screening, safety seminars, exercise and fitness programs, diet counseling, healthy eating, and stop-smoking programs.

Mind-Body Health: The study of the intersection of thought, attitudes, emotions, belief, and health/illness. Examples of mind-body health studies include coursework on health psychology, transpersonal psychology, mind-body medicine, holistic

Katherine Bracey Lorenzo is Professor of Psychology at Macomb Community College, Michigan.

nursing, global healing belief and practice, health and healing study groups, seminars, conferences, or special events dealing with the effects of positive thought, hypnosis, and the use of prayer in medicine.

The survey materials also differentiated between degree and non-degree programs and courses. While each of these delivery systems assumes an equally important educational role, the survey sought information as to which was more active in and/or responsive to the area of mind-body health education.

RESPONSES TO THE SURVEY

A total of 427 responses (both degree and non-degree) was received from 313 institutions. This was considered a gratifying response — significantly higher than anticipated. In 114 instances, colleges returned both forms; one from their academic divisions and one from continuing education or community services.

In the degree credit area. . . of the 313 responding institutions, 237 responses were completed and returned by the college's degree credit curriculum. Of these, 155 reported no mind-body health offerings. Of the remaining eighty-two, twenty-four institutions reported programs or courses that are *totally* mind-body health oriented. Fifty-eight institutions reported that they had degree credit offerings that were *partially* mind-body health oriented; that is, mind-body health was the focus of a small part of their degree credit curriculum. Eleven institutions reported that they offered mind-body health survey courses (general overviews of a theoretical nature) such as *Holistic Health* at Southeast Community College, NE and *Psychology of Health: Mind-Body Interaction* at Macomb Community College, MI. All others were health enhancement or skill teaching courses, such as meditation or yoga.

All of the nursing programs cited in the responses were either totally or partially mind-body oriented. In some cases, entire nursing programs were labeled *holistic,* such as that at Northern Maine Technical College where "both wellness and mind-body paradigms are woven throughout the two years of study."

Of note: Colleges reporting that they offered mind-body health classes in their degree credit curriculum areas experienced substantial interest in continuing and furthering their involvement in this field.

In the non-degree credit area. . . of the 313 responding institutions, 190 responses were completed and returned by the colleges' non-degree curriculum areas. Of these, ninety-five, or fifty percent, did offer mind-body health courses. Thirty-five were mind-body health education — explanations of what mind-body health is and how it "works" — while the balance addressed treatment modalities or ways to create mind-body health such as tai chi or yoga. The variety of offerings in this area was remarkably broad, with classes ranging from *Psycho-neuroimmunology and Aging*, offered by the City College of San Francisco, CA, to *Holistic Health: Body, Mind, Spirit* offered by Anne Arundel Community College, MD, to *Mind and Healing* offered by Clark College, WA, and to *Spirituality in the Treatment Setting*, offered by Edison Community College, OH.

Many non-degree classes addressed *alternative medicine* or *alternative healing techniques*, with homeopathy, herbal medicine, therapeutic talk, and massage therapy being the most popular. The most extensive offering was massage therapy, which reflected offerings in a broad variety of formats from workshops to complete certificate programs requiring up to 1,200 hours of instruction at Alvin Community College, TX and Grant MacEwan Community College, Canada.

Of note: Mind-body health education programs offered through non-degree credit classes are more numerous and diverse than those offered for degree credit. In fact, it is difficult to find two colleges with the same offerings since community service or continuing education departments are especially reliant on the local population's supply of instructors.

SELECTED QUOTATIONS FROM THE SURVEY RESPONSES

The following is a representative sampling of responses to queries regarding future plans and interest in the field of mind-body health on the part of the community colleges that returned survey forms.

- Since this is a field of evolving importance, we will give serious consideration to the development of a mind-body degree/certificate program.
  Dr. Hugh Craft, Dean, Nunez Community College, Chalmette, LA

- There is increasing interest in this area at our college and the possibility for developing more classes of this type certainly exists.
  Carolyn M. Allred, Department Head, Health and Physical Education, Central Piedmont Community College, Charlotte, NC

- We expect to develop a two-track mind-body program for Fall 1995. A professional series will be offered in addition to our personal enrichment courses. There is a growing interest in this area in our community.
  Andrew Meyer, Dean, CE/Extended Learning Programs, Anne Arundel Community College, Arnold, MD

- We plan to start a mind-body program next year in cooperation with our community wellness council.

  Elizabeth Stevens, Dean of Instruction, Sheridan College, Sheridan, NY

- Credit offerings are likely to be initiated in the future since interest in mind-body health is high in our non-credit courses.

  G.O. Kelly, Ph.D., President, Grant MacEwan Community College, Edmonton, Alberta

- We anticpate an increased demand in mind-body health courses; however, the current Regent's policy of little or no funding for this area will prohibit growth.

  Dr. Bill Sutterfield, Executive Vice-President, Tulsa Junior College, Tulsa, OK

- We have plans to offer *Principles of Healing* and a massage class in 1996.

  Julie Crutchfield, Division Chair, Health, Physical Education, Recreation, Scottsdale Community College, Scottsdale, AZ

- We are very interested and would like to see mind-body health classes increase.

  Arlene Jurgens, Chair, Nursing Department, Clackamas Community College, Oregon City, OR

- We have no plans at present, but would be very interested in what others are doing.

  Dr. John Y. Reid, Rowan-Cabarrus Community College, Salisbury, NC

- Mind-body programs are being considered. We need more information! Perhaps you can tell us about institutions with successful programs.

  W.E. Boggs, Administrative Assistant, Itawamba Community College, Fulton, MS

- We will be looking at mind-body health courses to replace or modify our current offerings.

  Dave Norfolk, Director, Continuing Education, Boston College, Muskogee, OK

- I anticipate that within the next five years our college will pilot some mind-body offerings.

  Barbara Thomason, Continuing Education Coordinator, Montgomery College, Conroe, TX

- We anticipate that mind-body studies will continue to grow as a strong program trend, with related offerings growing in number.

    Rita Martinez-Purson, Dean, Community Studies, Santa Fe Community College, Santa Fe, NM

- We expect mind-body offerings and enrollment to increase. There seems to be more public awareness of mind-body health issues.

    Janet M. Birnkrant, Director, Program Development, Kingsborough Community College, Brooklyn, NY

- Our open campus will continue to offer a variety of mind-body topics and subjects depending on demand, based on what the public will support. We are located in a rather traditional Bible-belt area, and are taking an introduction of these programs slowly.

    Donna George, Director, Institute of Human Development, Manatee Community College, Open Campus, Bradenton, FL

- Interest in mind-body programs continues to grow. We will certainly maintain our current offerings, and we anticipate some increase.

    Reva Shapiro, Director, Community Services, Brookdale Community College, Lincroft, NJ

- We expect an increase in the area of mind-body health studies.

    Kathy Hughes, (Dir. CE), Flathead Valley Community College, Kalispell, OR

- We anticipate a tremendous increase in the demand for these offerings. An example of this imminent increase is our magnetic touch healing class in Fall 1994; one third of the participants were health professionals (RNs and a PT) sent by Kaiser Permanente.

    Alexandra Au, Health Program Coordinator, Kapi'olani Community College, Honolulu, HI

- Our program of continuing education for health professionals will be expanding our course offerings related to mind-body alternative health care.

    Estelle Yahes, Coordinator, Continuing Education for Health Professionals, Rockland Community College, Suffern, NY

- We are planning a course for nursing professionals in which CEUs would be awarded. . . I anticipate that we will probably offer a non-credit mind-body health course at least once a year.

    Debbie Lovingood, Coordinator, Continuing Education, Madisonville Community College, Madisonville, KY

- Our college is in the process of expanding its continuing education program. Mind-body studies will be one of the areas considered for CEU offerings.

  Chris Laffer, Dean of Extended Services, Northeast State Technical and Community College, Blountville, TN

- I anticipate an increase in interest in mind-body health, and therefore a much broader spectrum of offerings through our non-credit program.

  Nancy Shepard, San Juan College, Farmington, NM

- Our health and wellness series is both professional development and personal enrichment. . . certificates are available. . . I see it expanding tremendously.

  Beverly Blue, Director, Comm. Health/Life Enhancement Institute, Delta College, Univ. Center, MI

The above constitutes a summary of the survey responses. Copies of the full survey report are available. Contact Diane U. Eisenberg at (202) 393-2208.

Part V

MIND-BODY HEALTH RESOURCES

ORGANIZATIONS

American Holistic Health Association
P. O. Box 17400
Anaheim, CA 92817
(714) 779-6152
Nonprofit educational organization that promotes a proactive,
holistic approach to health.

The Center for Mind-Body Medicine
5225 Connecticut Avenue, NW
Suite 414
Washington, D.C. 20015
(202) 966-7338
Educational health care program grounded in an appreciation of
the interpenetration of life's biological, psychological, spiritual,
and social dimensions.

Fetzer Institute
9292 West KL Avenue
Kalamazoo, MI 49009
(616) 375-2000
Nonprofit, private operating foundation promoting research
into health care methods that utilize the principles of mind-body
phenomena.

Institute of Noetic Sciences
475 Gate Five Road
Suite 300, Department M
Sausalito, CA 94966-0909
(800) 383-1394
Research, education and membership organization that includes
mind-body health among its interests. Co-produced TBS cable
television series *The Heart of Healing.*

National Community College
Wellness Conference
Contact: Elaine Sullivan, Richland College
2929 Marsann Lane
Farmers Branch
Dallas, Texas 75234
(214) 243-5333
An annual conference, conducted by community college faculty
and administrators, dedicated to the pursuit of mind-body
health and its implications for community colleges.

National Institute for the
Clinical Application of Behavioral Medicine
Box 523
Mansfield Center, CT 06250
(203) 456-1153
Provides practitioner-oriented conferences and seminars for
health care providers, specifically on the interface between
health and psychology.

National Institutes of Health
Office of Alternative Medicine
6120 Executive Blvd.
Suite 450
Rockville, MD 20892-9904
(301) 402-2466
Established in 1992, this Congressionally created federal center
evaluates and validates the most promising unconventional
medical practices.

Stress Reduction Clinic
University of Massachusetts Medical Center
55 Lake Avenue North
Worcester, MA 01655-0001
(508) 856-1616
Programs for patients and the training of health professionals.
Basic patient program in mindfulness meditation and its
applications for living with stress, pain, and chronic illness.

Books

Encounters with Qi:
Exploring Chinese Medicine
David Eisenberg. New York: Penguin Books, 1987.
An American doctor's observations in China of the use of qi
(pronounced chi) or "vital energy"—the unifying principle of
Chinese medicine.

Full Catastrophe Living: Using the Wisdom of Body & Mind to Face Stress, Pain & Illness
Jon Kabat-Zinn. New York: Delacorte Press, 1990.
Based on the successful program for patients with stress-related
disorders and chronic pain the author directs at the University of
Massachusetts Medical Center.

Healing and the Mind
Bill Moyers. New York: Doubleday, 1993.
A companion to the public television series of the same name,
this best-seller features interviews with experts in the field of
mind-body health.

The Heart of Healing
Institute of Noetic Sciences with William Poole. Atlanta:
Turner Publishing, 1993.
This companion to the television series goes around the world
to examine how research, clinical practice, and patient experiences
are validating mind-body connections.

Living Beyond Limits: New Hope and Help for Facing Life-Threatening Illness
David Spiegel. New York: Times Books, 1994.
Focusing on the author's landmark study of women with breast cancer, this book discusses how people with serious illness live longer, fuller lives when medical treatment is joined by psychosocial support.

Mind/Body Medicine: How To Use Your Mind For Better Health
Daniel Goleman and Joel Gurin, eds.
Yonkers, NY: Consumer Reports, 1993.
(914) 398-2000
Guide to mind-body health that combines a review of the research with practical advice. Chapters by leading experts in the field.

Minding the Body, Mending the Mind
Joan Borysenko. Toronto: Bantam Books, 1988.
Drawing on the latest findings in mind-body research, this book demonstrates that many common ailments can often be improved or completely corrected without drugs or invasive medical procedures.

Stress Management
James S. Gordon. New York: Chelsea House Publishers, 1990.
Traces the interaction between stress and bodily functions and describes a few of the programs available to manage the condition.

Where the Mind Meets the Body
Harris Dienstfrey. New York: HarperCollins Publishers, 1992.
An introductory overview that examines modalities by which the mind can be used to improve physical health. Also addresses the conscious and unconscious dimension of the mind-body interaction.

PERIODICALS

Advances: The Journal of Mind-Body Health
Fetzer Institute
9292 West KL Avenue
Kalamazoo, MI 49009
(616) 375-2000
A quarterly journal that reports developments in the study of mind-body health and explores their implications for health care, medical training, and further research.

Common Boundary
Common Boundary, Inc.
Charles H. Simpkinson, Ph.D., Publisher.
430 East-West Highway
Bethesda, MD 20814
(301) 652-9495
A bimonthly magazine that explores the relationship between
psychology and spirituality.

Mental Medicine Update
Institute for the Study of Human Knowledge
David Sobel, M.D. and
Robert Ornstein, Ph.D., eds.
P.O. Box 176
Los Altos, CA 94023
(415) 948-9428
Newsletter focusing on the effects of mood, personality, social support,
and other psychosocial factors in health. Intended to help bridge the gaps
between mind and body, research and practice, patient and professional.

AUDIOTAPES

Roots of Healing: The New Medicine
Michael Toms and Andrew Weil.
New Dimensions Radio, 1994.
(415) 563-8899
This series of three one-hour audiotapes explores topics such as
psychospiritual approaches to healing in life-threatening illness,
and how patients can take further responsibility for their own care.

Beyond Cure: Four Talks on Healing for Health Professionals
Rachel Naomi Remen, M.D.
Institute for the Study of Health and Illness at Commonweal.
(415) 868-2245
In these hour-long lectures, the director of the Institute explores the
creative use of illness and provides a new perspective on the
psychological process in ill people.

VIDEOTAPES

Healing and the Mind With Bill Moyers
Ambrose Video Publishing
1290 Avenue of the Americas
New York, NY 10104
(800) 843-0048 for home orders
(800) 526-4663 for institutional orders
In this award-winning, five-part public television series, Bill Moyers explores the connections between mind, body and spirit.

The Heart of Healing
Time-Life Video
(800) 621-7026
This revised, eight-part version of the TBS documentary series focuses on people and communities across the world and shows how research, clinical practice, and patient experiences are validating mind-body connections.

The Meaning of Health:
A Dialogue With Bill Moyers
Mystic Fire Video
PO Box 2249
Livonia, MI 48151
(800) 292-9001
An expanded, philosophical exploration of ideas generated by *Healing and the Mind With Bill Moyers*, this video features a roundtable discussion among some of the principal experts featured in the public television series.

Part VI

PARTICIPANTS: MIND-BODY HEALTH COMMUNITY COLLEGE ROUNDTABLE

MARCH 14-15, 1995

SEASONS: A CENTER FOR RENEWAL
FETZER INSTITUTE
KALAMAZOO, MICHIGAN

Anne Benvenuti
Dean, Kern Valley Campus
Cerro Coso Community College
P.O. Box 1447
Kernville, CA 93238

John J. Cavan
President
Southside Virginia Community College
R.R. 1, Box 60
Alberta, VA 23821

Barry S. Eisenberg
Conference Reporter
Mind-Body Health Community College Roundtable
444 North Capitol St. NW, Suite 428
Washington, DC 20001

Diane U. Eisenberg
Project Director
Mind-Body Health Community College Roundtable
444 North Capitol St. NW, Suite 428
Washington, DC 20001

Joel Elkes
Senior Scholar in Residence and Fetzer Fellow
1712 Glenhouse Drive
Apt. 417, Pelican Cove
Sarasota, FL 34231

James S. Ford
Chair, Mind-Body Health Program
Professor, Psychology
Community College of Aurora
16000 East Centretech Parkway
Aurora, CO 80011-9036

Jack Fujimoto
President *(on assignment)*
Educational Development/ Governmental Relations
Los Angeles Community College District
770 Wilshire Boulevard
Los Angeles, CA 90017

James S. Gordon
Fetzer Fellow
Director
The Center for Mind-Body Medicine
5225 Connecticut Avenue, NW, Suite 414
Washington, DC 20015

Edward Haring
Vice President for Instruction
Kellogg Community College
450 North Avenue
Battle Creek, MI 49016

Albert Lorenzo
President
Macomb Community College
14500 Twelve Mile Road
Warren, MI 48093

Katherine Bracey Lorenzo
Professor, Psychology
Macomb Community College
44575 Garfield, B-114
Clinton Township, MI 48038

James Mahoney
Director, Academic, Student, and International Services
American Association of Community Colleges
One Dupont Circle, Suite 410
Washington, DC 20036

Mickey Olivanti
Program Associate
Fetzer Institute
9292 West KL Avenue
Kalamazoo, MI 49009

Esther Perantoni
Program Developer, Continuing Education
Northern Virginia Community College
Loudon Campus
1000 Harry Byrd Highway
Sterling, VA 20164

David Sluyter
Program Director
Fetzer Institute
9292 West KL Avenue
Kalamazoo, MI 49009

Elaine Sullivan
Representative
National Community College Wellness Conference
Richland College
12800 Abrams Road
Dallas, TX 75243

James Turcott
Instructor of Psychology
Kalamazoo Valley Community College
6767 West O Avenue
Kalamazoo, MI 49009

Molly Vass
Fetzer Fellow
Director of the Holistic Healthcare Program
Western Michigan University
B-314 Ellsworth
Kalamazoo, MI 49008

Shannon Whitten
Student
Brevard Community College
731 Whispering Pines Circle
Melbourne, FL 32940

Part VII

COMMENTS FROM
ROUNDTABLE PARTICIPANTS

"As economic pressures for higher productivity continually increase, mind-body health offers the best antidote to maintain the health and humanity of the American workforce."

> — James S. Ford
> Chair, Mind-Body Health Center
> Professor, Psychology
> Community College of Aurora

"Because of its long-standing commitment to enhancing individual and community well-being, the community college is the logical choice to further public under-standing of the principles of mind-body health."

> — Albert L. Lorenzo
> President
> Macomb Community College

"It certainly is appropriate that democracy's colleges, the institutions that made higher education an egalitarian right, be the delivery system for mind-body health studies. Providing all Americans with this type of education will give them better control of their lives, providing a better quality of life for individuals and more productivity for society."

> — John J. Cavan
> President
> Southside Virginia Community College

"Community colleges are well positioned to educate their students and community members to the broad spectrum of health and healing approaches."

—   Shannon Whitten
        Student
        Brevard Community College

"The PBS series *Healing and the Mind with Bill Moyers* resulted in a tremendous upsurge in community interest in the topic. Mind-body health education seems like a natural intersect with the role of the community college. There is a readiness for this kind of teaching. We see the interest everywhere."

—   David Sluyter
        Program Director
        Fetzer Institute

"In our quest to understand our physical environment, physics has produced a concept called 'field theory.' This concept explains how one physical entity can affect another physical entity with only empty space between the two. Field theory as an explanation for gravitational and electromagnetic interactions is openly explored, used and widely accepted. Why then is it so difficult or uncomfortable for us to explore a mind-body connection?"

—   Edward Haring
        Vice President for Instruction
        Kellogg Community College

"How appropriate that mind-body health be an intrinsic part of the learning process through the nation's community colleges."

—   Esther Perantoni
        Program Developer, Continuing Education
        Northern Virginia Community College,
                Loudon Campus

"Community colleges are in a position to foster wholeness in the lives of individuals in communities throughout the United States."

—   Molly Vass
        Director of the Holistic Healthcare Program
        Western Michigan University

"Since 1988 a group of community college leaders have been designing and hosting an annual National Community College Wellness Conference dedicated to the pursuits of mind-body health and its implications in community colleges. We are enthused by AACC's leadership and commitment to the continued growth of mind-body health education as evidenced by this publication."

> — Elaine M. Sullivan
> Representative
> National Community College Wellness Conference

"I believe there is an urgent need for accurate, affordable, and appropriate mind-body health education and that the community college is uniquely suited to be the vehicle to bring that instruction to the waiting community."

> — Katherine Bracey Lorenzo
> Professor, Psychology
> Macomb Community College

"In terms of behaviors, skills, knowledge and attitudes, the changes needed in health care's emphasis and treatment must be brought about by educational efforts. People must be taught the value and importance of primary responsibility for their own health. People must be introduced to knowledge of their own requirements for well-being. People must be trained in the skills needed to actually care for themselves. These are all educational endeavors. The question now at hand is "Where will people acquire this knowledge and these skills?" And the best answer is "At their local community college," because the community college is available to everyone, has facilities and well-qualified staff already in place, and, most importantly has as its historical mission the education of adults."

> — Anne Benvenuti
> Dean, Kern River Valley Campus
> Cerro Coso College

"It is very important for community college students to have access to mind-body health, to help them cope with stress in their daily lives."

> — Jack Fujimoto
> President *(on assignment)*
> Educational Development/Governmental Relations
> Los Angeles Community College District